MOLDING A MIGHTY GRIP

by
George F. Jowett

DISCLAIMER

The exercises and advice contained within this book is for educational and entertainment purposes only. The exercises described may be too strenuous or dangerous for some people, and the reader should consult with a physician before engaging in any of them.

The author and publisher of this book are not responsible in any manner whatsoever for any injury, which may occur through the use or misuse of the information presented here.

Molding A Mighty Grip originally published in the 1930.

Manufactured in the United States of America

MOLDING A MIGHTY GRIP

BY

GEORGE F. JOWETT

Molding a Mighty Grip

By **GEORGE F. JOWETT**

D id you ever try to lift a keg of nails and carry it, free of the body, by grasping the keg by the chines? The next opportunity you get I wish you would try it. You might be surprised with the results. A keg of nails weighs anywhere from 100 lbs. up, but to check up on yourself the 100-lb. keg will be sufficient. In order to lift this unwieldy object you will be obliged to lay it on its side. The only grip the chines will afford will be that secured by the first joint of the fingers – the finger tips. If you lift the barrel free of the body the lift will be sustained purely by the strength of the fingers, which will be the index to how much grip you really have.

Most people labor under the belief that a strong grip is the result of a big pair of biceps, or a huge pair of forearms. Biceps have nothing to do with a strong grip and while large forearms can have a great deal to do with a powerful grip, yet this depends largely upon how the forearms were developed and which muscles in the forearm are best developed. This statement may surprise you somewhat but perhaps you have never given much thought to the fact that there are nineteen muscles which go to make up the constructive bulk of the forearm. Of these nineteen muscles *only four* are concerned with the pronator and supinator movements. I wish you to remember this as a probable answer to you forearm developing problems; simply because the general trend of forearm exercises is centered around these four – and, as a more positive fact I might say that these muscles are not generally sufficiently treated. Nine of the nineteen muscles control the movements of the thumb and finger and six govern the wrist.

As you will now readily understand there are more muscles governing the finger and the wrist movements than most exercise fans realize. A checkup on this is proven by an inventory of your stock of forearm exercises. They will be few, but the number of exercises advocated and practiced for the wrist and the fingers will be even less. It is for the reason that I wanted to prove to you the absence of the

3

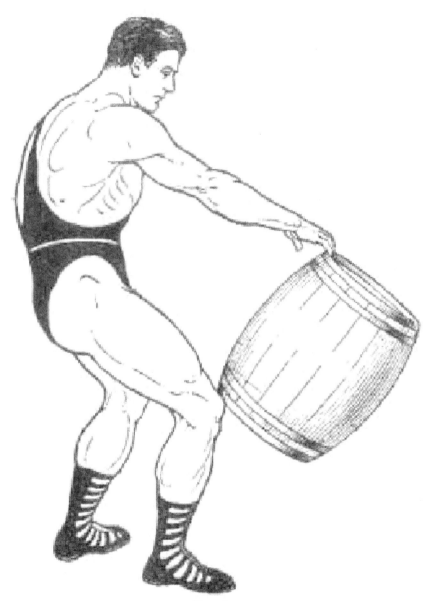

FIG. 1

test your ability on the keg of nails. It may prove an unusual test for you but a very effective one.

With the old-time strong man, tossing around nail kegs and barrels filled with water was a favorite method of demonstrating his strength. In fact, such tests often comprised the entire set of feats in deciding a strength contest. The feats were not confined to the mere lifting of the keg or barrel off the floor by grasping the chines. The test were varied, such as lifting clear of the floor, lifting in one clean movement onto the thighs, then in one or two movements to the shoulders and another method is to sweep the keg or barrel from the floor to arm's length overhead in one clean movement. In all of these tests remember the only grip allowed is that secured by the fingers upon the chines of the keg or barrel.

The French-Canadians have a very difficult barrel feat, which, if you are proud of your grip and arm strength, you ought to try. The barrel is tipped forward and the nearest edge of the barrel is brought to rest upon the thigh just above the knee – a part of the feat made easier by bending the knee well forward. You grasp the barrel chine nearest and perform the first part of the stunt as illustrated in Fig. 1. The next movement is to quickly pull the barrel toward you and lie back to counterbalance the pull. As the barrel passes the perpendicular point of balance it will quickly fall toward the body. You must then quickly let go you hand grip on the chine and receive the barrel at the shoulder.

Louis Cyr, the famous Canadian strong man and, incidentally, the man considered by all the leading strong men of yesterday and today to be the strongest man that ever lived, was phenomenally mighty in this particular feat. The combination water and sand filled barrel that he was able to shoulder with one hand, was of a weight nigh unbelievable. August Johnson, the European champion strong man of those days, was also a physical giant in handling barrels. When he and Cyr clashed for the honor of the world's title, barrel feats were important features of the contest. In Johnson, Cyr met a foeman worthy of his steel – it brought out the best that was in the great Canadian, and it was needed in order to conclusively defeat this splendid European strength athlete – which Cyr did. Barrels ranging from 300 pounds to

500 pounds were tossed around in that long journey of strength. Cyr gripped and lifted slippery chines until his fingers bled. It was a battle of giants in which the true caliber of muscle and endurance was tested to the limit. When one recalls the strength contests of those days thaat lasted hours, it makes one smile at the three and four lift contests of today.

Johnson and Cyr were men famous for the tremendous grip, hand and finger power each had. Each possessed as fine an arm in size and contour as ever hung on a man and their wrists were deep with steel-like sinews. These men, like many others, practiced exercises involving the use of the fingers and hand grip equally as much as they did the other muscular members, which is the reason for their all-round physical strength. Of late years strength athletes have mostly confined themselves to the few standard lifts – the old feats and exercises are not practiced, or are forgotten. This, and no other reason, explains why so few strong athletes, no matter how good they are at overhead lifts, have little better than an ordinary grip. It must, of course, be understood, overhead lifting does not involve the necessity of a grip of steel. In fact, the grip is only necessary at the commencement of a lift when the weight is taken from off the floor in starting it to the shoulder. The grip must be quick to get the start, then instantly relaxed, otherwise it would interfere with the rest of the lift.

The introduction of lifting with a free or open grip in this country is credited to me. This type of grip certainly improved the records of the many strength athletes I have taught. To develop the enviable grip of steel you must do the things which create it and above all you must know the right muscles to develop and not waste time on other exercises which apparently stimulate the grip, but actually do not. Do not waste time on such movements as only employ what grip you have – they are not developing movements. There is a great difference. In this connection there is often the same misunderstanding as is frequently found in the selection of arm exercises. Many exercises call for a great tension of the arm muscles, but that is all. Tension will not aid muscular growth, it merely employs what you have, it keeps the effort centered in one place only. In order to aid growth full muscular operation must be increased. All possible extension and contraction must be provided by the exercise, then results will begin to show.

I think the reason why a lot of tensing exercises are favored is because the exerciser has been taught to believe the longer a muscle effort is sustained the better results he will obtain. This is only true as far as the extension and contraction of muscle is involved but it must be remembered that all muscles have different lengths and must be estimated accordingly. The important thing to remember about the forearm muscle is that they are, with the exception of one, all short-range muscles, particularly those which influence the movements of the wrist and fingers. This fact should inspire the grip and arm developer to dig in, as it means less exhaustive exercises but exercises in which greater concentration can be employed with a vast saving in energy.

No doubt you will have noticed that invariably all hand balancers have splendidly-formed arms and each has a firm, powerful hand clasp. I have found that hand balancers on the whole have a more perfectly-formed arm – particularly the forearms and wrist – than the weight lifter. The hand balancer employs the hand and wrist much more than does the lifter of weights and what is more interesting, he employs the arm muscles as well as the grip in many unusual ways – ways not possible to the exercise fans who handle weights only. No doubt knowledge of this diversified method of development is what makes the mass of European strength athletes so partial to the practice of hand balancing. The average American strength athlete could practice this valuable pastime of hand balancing more consistently than he does.

Above all else, hand balancing requires a very strong and flexible wrist, it requires you to be able to bend the hand back on the forearm greatly. To do this further extension of the muscles that form on the front of the forearm is necessary. If you are not adept at making, and holding, a balance standing on the hands you will quickly become acquainted with the feeling of a great pressure upon the wrist – later the wrist will feel very stiff. Naturally part of this is caused by the wrists trying to support the body weight, but the main cause is that the forearm muscles, and those of the wrist and the hand, are exerting themselves unusually in helping to attain, and retain, your balance in the hand stand. Every hand balancer will recognize the truth of what I have just written.

Many exercise fans find it very difficult to perform certain wrist movements, but hand balancers rarely find any wrist movements difficult. Constant practice in juggling their body weight upon their hands develops for them remarkable hand control. Usually they are adepts in the interesting practice of "wrist turning," a sport in which the combination of hand grip, wrist flexibility and arm power are the chief assets. This sport has always been one of my pet strength testing pastimes and at this sport I have turned wrists with all the great celebrities in most every country for many years.

As I recall, the earliest practice I adopted for strengthening my hand and wrist for this sport was to take a fairly heavy spring. In one end I drove a round piece of wood to serve as a handle. The other end I fastened to a bench. I would grasp the wooden handle with one hand and by keeping the elbow close to the bench would seek, by forearm strength alone, to bend the spring over until the wooden handle touched the bench. This exercise I would repeat a number of times and then change over to the other hand. As I grew stronger I increased the size and strength of the spring until I got so that very few of the strongest men were able to do much with the spring I could force down. I loved to feel my muscles quiver with the resistance. The practice stood me in good stead during my wrestling career, and I know anyone will benefit materially if he includes a little of this for grip and arm developing. It is a simple thing which anyone can rig up.

The hands present a very interesting study. It is often stated they reflect your physical characteristics equally as much as the face. It is quite true the grip is the barometer of a certain amount of your physical strength and the energy you possess – though many carry the grip business to extremes. Some do not know the difference between a firm hand clasp and wringing the hand of an acquaintance like a dish rag. Judgment should be used no matter how strong your grip is. Remember, every one admires a firm grip but no one has any desire to present his hand for a pulp crushing demonstration.

MOLDING A MIGHTY GRIP

Hands are as varied in construction as are the builds of different people. Some have long, slender, tapering hands; others have big hands and long fingers, big hands and short fingers, thick hands, small hands, sinewy hands and heavy hands. It is impossible to say which of these is the best. I have seen hands, of every construction named here, possessed of remarkable strength.

A big hand does not always indicate a big arm. We have such men as Moerki and Inch having unusually small hands but it would be extremely difficult to find men with superior gripping power. Many exercise fans have told me they know they cannot build a powerful arm and grip because they possess small hands. Personally, I do not think this should enter into the subject at all, because when all is said and done it is the muscles that count. It is a common belief that because of having a small wrist and hand, enough power cannot be produced to develop the muscles. As a matter of fact the rotating and twisting movement of the hand is produced, not at the wrist joint, but by the crossing of the bones of the forearm. The bones of the forearm are so united that one of them may rotate around the other. This bone movement increases the utility of the hand. By this means we are enabled to perform such acts as inserting a corkscrew or turning a screwdriver.

These two bones are named the *radius* and the *ulna*. It is the shaft of the *radius* that passes obliquely across the front of the shaft of the *ulna*. When the arm is in the prone position, with the palm directed downwards, we can reverse the action and bring the palm upwards again. This is the movement of supination. Pronation and supination therefore are movements whereby we may rotate the axis of the hand through an arc of 180 degrees, or about half a circle.

It is a point worthy of consideration that a considerable number of the muscles lodged in the forearm, whilst indirectly controlling the movements of the wrist, are in their main action directly concerned with the movements of the fingers. It will be at once apparent that had accommodation for all these muscles, which act on the fingers, been provided in the hand itself, it would have involved a great increase in the size and bulk of the member, since the space required to lodge the

9

muscular fibres necessary to generate the force required, would be considerable. To obviate this, nature has adopted the ingenious plan of placing the fleshy bellies of these muscles in the forearm and arranging for the transmission of the force to the moving parts by means of a series of long, slender tendons, which are easily accommodated at the wrist and take up but little room. In this way the tapering form of the arm, which is small in the region of the wrist and of great bulk higher up where the fleshy bellies of those muscles are situated, is easily accounted for. A small wrist would therefore indicate that the muscle which form the front of the forearm are poorly developed. This is usually the case, even with many persistent exercisers.

The muscular construction on the front of the forearm is not proportionate with the back. The muscles on the front of your forearm are really your gripping muscles. It is common knowledge that the flexor movements of the wrist and fingers are more powerful than the extensor actions. For this reason it should be quite obvious that the flexor muscles in the front of the arm can be more strongly developed than the muscles which lie on the back of the forearm associated with the extensor movements.

Examine the forearm development of as many muscle builders as you come in contact with and you will see that if development in the front of the forearm is lacking theses people are not nearly so capable at gripping and arm strength as the muscle builders who have thoroughly developed the front of the forearm.

If you clench the fingers tightly and bend the hand down on the front of the forearm – shortening the distance between the hand and the elbow – you will clearly see how much developed are your gripping muscles. With many this demonstration will not change the contour of the front forearm, with some others a small knot of muscle becomes apparent just below the elbow.

What is required is a sweeping line commencing from the wrist and bulging powerfully as the line ascends to the elbow. Pictures of forearm development are very deceiving. I recall a certain strength athlete being especially written up as having a marvelous development.

I happened to be very well acquainted with this athlete and knew that by measurements he was away below many others I knew, also that he is inferior in gripping strength, but he looked good because he had a small wrist. His forearm is almost a straight line halfway down the arms and then it suddenly bulges forward into what looks like a huge lump of muscle. The gripping muscles, by some freak of nature, were only partially developed whereas they should be moulded from wrist to elbow. Study the forearms of Zottman, Joe Nordquest and Jim Pedley and you will see the difference.

It has been said that I possess one of the finest sets of developed gripping muscles seen. It is true that at one time my wrist size was only average but as the gripping muscles increased in size so did my wrist size increase. My hand is very powerful looking and broad, the fingers are short but very sinewy and the setting of the thumb on the hand is unusual, being like a big hook which is what has given my hand powerful forcep thumb action. You must not forget that the fingers provide the hand with gripping and clenching action but the different muscular construction of the thumb provides the hand with forcep power which is not possible to the fingers, excepting the small finger in a minor degree; consequently, in all pinching efforts the thumb is the most powerful factor, aided slightly by the little finger. Despite all this, the middle finger is capable of lifting more weight off the floor than when all the fingers and the thumb are employed. This is due to its location on the hand.

If you study the various illustrations in this book of the hand, wrist and forearm you will see, without my going into lengthy detail, exactly how the muscles are ordered and how they influence the wrist, hand and fingers. I would rather devote the space to exercise explanations and stunts that will give you the fabled grip of steel.

Personally, I think there are more interesting methods to choose from for developing a mighty grip than are possible for developing any other particular set of muscles. Of course, I realize many of these methods may not be known to you as most of them have not been introduced in America, though the strength athletes of prewar days were somewhat familiar with some of them. I have in the past written many articles on these methods which originated mostly in Canada and Europe and judging from the many letters I received it was quite apparent if more such articles had been written those methods would have been intensely popular over here. I learned them when I was abroad in my early professional days and from contact with such iron arm specialists as Marx, Pedley, Vanstittart, De Carrie and many others.

Of course, exercises alone are a good way of developing the grip and forearm muscles but I have always believed that exercises which are more of the stunt type give better results. The exercises then become more interesting. They make one adept, at the same time they increase the grip and muscular size. It is also more interesting to be able to perform competitive feats among your friends when such can be done without the use of cumbersome apparatus. You are apt to practice more often and you will certainly get more kick out of it. Juggling a 50-pound block weight is full of interest, fun and grip development. I practiced this sport all my life and used to give many interesting exhibitions with a block weight. You will be amazed how your grip and arms will respond to this interesting practice. When purchasing a block weight get one that is absolutely square and compact. A block weight oblong in shape from the handle down is far too awkward to handle. Some mighty feats can be performed with a block weight. It is one practice which affords an opportunity to prove how much thumb forcep power you have. One of my best stunts is to use a pinch grip with the thumb and index finger on the bar and pick a 50-pound block weight up as high as my shoulders. Some hook the finger round the bar, but that makes it easy. Just try it my way and you will readily realize why few are able to do it. As a matter of fact, I have never seen anyone do it correctly though I do not doubt Marx, Saxon and Vanstittart could do it.

Before I pass on I wish to say that it is not necessary that you definitely use a 50-lb. block weight. You will probably find it too much, therefore, get a block weight within your power, for it is better to practice correctly with an object well within your ability than to struggle with one that taxes your strength to the limit.

Gripping an iron disc between finger and thumb is great for

developing the grip and forcep power of the thumb. Generally speaking a person is acknowledged to be very strong in the hand to be able to raise a plate weighing 75 lbs. A plate 1 inch thick is usually used. It is always best to start with a light weight and work up. Try, for a change, picking a plate up by the edge, using in progressive order the four fingers with the thumb, then three fingers and so on until only the index finger and thumb are employed.

One of the oldest tests of grip and arm strength is that of breaking horseshoes. When I was only a boy I used to frequent blacksmith shops and practice on discarded, worn-out shoes. It sure was great fun. I always looked forward to the day when I would be able to break apart a good sized brand new horseshoe. That day was a proud day for me. I would not then have changed places with a millionaire. John Marx was the daddy of 'em all at bending horseshoes. He could bend the largest shoe ever made to wear on a horse. In this act he regularly used a shoe that would withstand the efforts of ten or more men pulling in tug of war formation. After this he would bend the shoe without any noticeably great effort. He had the strength of grip, arm and shoulder that is seldom, if ever, equalled.

One time Professor Desbonnet had some special horsehoes that had been made just for the purpose of surprising some of the strong men who were likely to call on the professor and display their wares. When genial John Marx called at the Desbonnet School the professor was very pleased to have the big fellow try his hand on these shoes which had resisted others for years. Marx bent the shoes to the amazement of the professor and did it without any great physical exertion.

Picking up thick-handled iron bars is another grip-building stunt. You can quite often be stumped with a fairly light weight if your grip is not sufficient to grasp the thick handle. This has always been a pet stunt of the strong man. Noel, a very strong Frenchman, had a dumbell which weighed 110 lbs. He claimed no one except himself, no matter how quickly they tried to snap it up, could lift it to the shoulder with one hand, so large was the grip. He tried Marx out but got the shock of his life when the burly giant nonchalantly picked it up and even slowly curled it to the shoulder. Can you imagine doing a slow arm curl to the shoulder of 110 pounds with even a regular sized handle grip? Then how much more difficult must it have been with the thick handled grip.

George Zottman had an iron ball to be lifted with the hand grip alone which he liked to use to stump all strong men. You were obliged to spread the hand over the ball and actually were only able to lift it with the finger tips. Zottman had a huge hand and the ball was shaped to his hand. A friend took me down to see him and the stunt was suggested. I agreed to try but Zottman claimed my hand was too small; nevertheless, I lifted it and on that particular day Zottman was unable to do it.

Picking up billiard cues by the tip and holding them out on the line level with the shoulder is a feat that develops great hand strength. W.P. Casell was undefeatable at this stunt. He had a mighty grip and splendidly formed arms. He was great at lifting overhead a 200-pound bar bell using one finger of each hand, but at this my famous Canadian pupil, Fournier, could go one better. He could do 230 pounds any time, using only one finger of each hand.

Henry Holtgrewe, of Cincinnati, one of the strongest men this country ever had, was particularly good at the following combination arm and grip stunt:

Lay a straw broom on the floor and on the straw end place a brick. By grasping the handle of the broom at the extreme end you raise broom and brick off the floor keeping same in a direct line with the forearm.

Ottley Coulter is good at this feat. He said before he was able to duplicate the broom and brick stunt of Holtgrewe, he was able to tear telephone directories into fractions and chin himself by grasping the under side of rafters, which is some grip test. Of course, the thing to do is start off light and increase the weight as your strength increases. This stunt is a teaser for the wrists and, done as Holtgrewe and Coulter do it, it is one that stops many strength athletes who are exceptionally good at other body feats of strength.

One of the greatest feats of gripping strength which Arthur Saxon was capable of was to snatch from the ground to arm's length overhead with two hands a deal plank two inches thick, weighing 180 lbs. Just try an ordinary 12-inch board 12 feet long with an inch thickness. Stand it on its edge with the length running parallel with the feet, then with one movement snatch it off the ground to arm's length overhead. I doubt whether you will succeed. Being light it will give you, in a small way, some conception of the terrific hand grip of Arthur Saxon.

I never knew another man to be able to lift Saxon's board off the ground with his hand grip, let alone snatch it to arm's length overhead.

FINGER PULLING

Finger pulling is a very popular sport in the Swiss Tyrol. These sturdy mountaineers seem to be especially adapted for the sport. The contestants lock the middle fingers, as shown in the illustration, and then pull. If the pulling is done while standing up then the heaviest man has the advantage, but if the contestants sit opposite each other at a table the advantage of greater weight is somewhat minimized. If it be agreed between the contestants that the free hand can be used to push against the table, then the struggle is apt to be more vigorous, otherwise opponents of about the same weight are only fairly matched. If you can straighten out the finger of your opponent you will have proof of great finger strength. The middle finger has terrific resistance. It is the best member of the hand to do a finger lift with.

Adrian Schmidt is a marvel at this stunt. He weighs only 126 lbs. but can out pull on a finger pull a giant like Joe Nordquest.

His fingers are like steel pinions. Well, figure it out for yourself. He can chin himself using only the thumb and index finger in a pinch grip on the last link of a suspended chain. He is the only man I ever heard tell of who could do this feat. It sounds superhuman but I know Schmidt could do it when he was 58 years old. He certainly built his muscles and strength to stay with him.

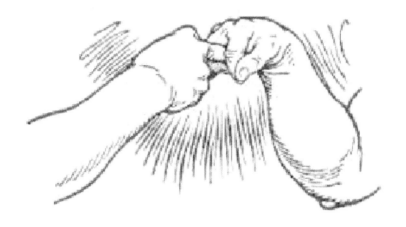

WRIST TURNING

Wrist turning is a true test of grip and arm strength. The object is to clasp hands in the manner shown, each with the elbow resting on top of a table. Each contestants is seated with the disengaged arm placed upon the table. The disengaged hand is not allowed to grasp the edge of the table. When the referee gives the word to "go" both the contestants must commence by slowly exerting their pressure. To try to get the jump on an opponent by snapping into action is not fair and no test of strength. The man who forces his opponent's hand down 3 out of 5 or 2 out of 3 times is adjudged the winner. Men with the front of the forearm well developed and with strong deltoids always excel at this sport. One of the toughest experiences I had in a wrist turning duel was with a French-Canadian lumberjack. He was not a real big man, but what a grip he had. It was like a vise. We both struggled like giants but finally I defeated him.

I have often been asked who afforded me the severest test in wrist turning. This is difficult to answer as I have contested with so many wonderful men who took all that was in me in order to win. Incidentally my best opponents were more or less unknown as strong men but were specialists in wrist turning.

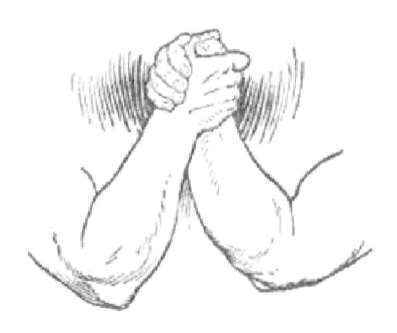

GEORGE F. JOWETT

EXERCISE ONE

The exercises in this book should all prove to be very interesting to every exercise fan. They savor so much of feats there is never a possibility of monotony. Take the exercise shown here, Exercise 1 (a). You will be surprised to find how weak the fingers will prove to be providing, of course, you use a book of fairly good weight. You will notice that the book is placed upon the fingers only and is not even touching the hand. Also note that the hand is not resting on the table. These two points are important. Naturally, you will understand you must use a book of sufficient weight but not so heavy as to make the exercise a strain. A straining movement has no value. It is the several properly executed movements that count. If you allow the back or the palm of the hand to rest on the table the major value of the exercise will be lost.

Notice how far the book is placed on the fingers and that the thumb has no part in the exercise. Your first effort will be to raise the volume as high as possible with the index finger as shown, Exercise 1 (b). When you have thus raised the book to your limit, lower back to the original position and employ the next finger and so on until every finger on both hands has exercised with the exception of the thumb. We will not miss the thumb – that comes later.

You may practice raising the book with each finger several times in succession before passing on ti its mate. This is really a better policy.

As you pass on the little finger you may find it somewhat difficult to juggle a book. The far side of the book may touch on the table, but do not let that worry you. It is perfectly all right as long as you feel the resistance.

When you have satisfactorily concluded the individual exercises, as just explained, try raising the book with the fingers one after the other, quickly, in the manner used to play a piano. This will create speed in your digits as well as strength.

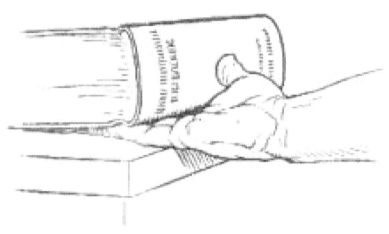

Exercise 1 (a)

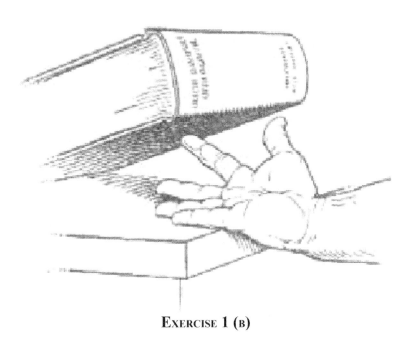

EXERCISE 1 (B)

Nimble as your fingers may be under ordinary circumstances you will find they will acquire an awkwardness when called upon to operate quickly and strongly as required in the piano movement.

If you have a volume sufficiently heavy you will find operating all the fingers of the hand at once a very good exercise also.

Finger exercises of all kinds have a very stimulating and gratifying influence upon developing the difficult muscles of the forearm which, at the same time, will naturally tend to increase the thickness of the wrist.

EXERCISE TWO

To practice this exercise you simply reverse the position of the hand with regard to the table as the illustration shows. This will be a little more difficult to some than to others, but you must not be dismayed, the exercise is not so difficult. This exercise will bring into action the forcep muscles of the thumb and of the little finger. As these two forcep factors operate you will notice the difference in both control and power. Control will be better and power more evident.

You go through the same process as explained for the first exercise, exercising the fingers individually and quickly in piano play fashion. The only action in this exercise requiring more care than in Exercise 1 is when the little finger becomes involved. As your fingers travel individually to the small finger a natural inclination will be felt to operate the thumb, commencing with the third finger and becoming more pronounced with the little finger. This last member has a certain amount of forcep action which, with the thumb, plays the major muscular action in closing the hand and gripping an object.

While what I am going to say now is a deviation from the subject yet it explains perhaps more clearly the importance wrestlers place upon the little finger in the self defense act against strangling. When a hand is gripped upon the throat the power of strangling is gotten most from the forceps action of the hand. The little finger does not cup the throat so well, therefore, when reaching for the strangling hands, the little fingers are easily got hold of and a quick down pull not only breaks the little finger hold but paralyzes the forearm power of the hand. This explains the dual connection and action of the little finger and thumb and the reason why, as the little finger comes into action, a natural inclination of the thumb to assist is felt in this exercise. Consequently, when the third finger becomes involved the thumb will be pushing strongly on the table as the little finger lifts. Cooperate with this double action by pushing down hard with the thumb as the little finger lifts.

There is another way of developing the finger and hand strength with which you probably are partly familiar. Done in the way I will outline it gives one, on first attempt, a feeling of lack of control and power in the arms. Nevertheless it will make your hand and finger strength increase greatly. The noticeable feature of this development will be in the finger sinews. They will become cordy and the fingers will gain suppleness, flexibility and speed. Suppose you try it.

The exercise is a chinning exercise performed exactly as you would chin a bar, the only difference being, instead of using a round bar you use a flat piece of wood. Place all the of the fingers flat on the board, and allow the thumb to remain free of the board. In this manner chin yourself several times. In order to make this exercise more progressive allow less of the finger space to hold on the board.

As a boy I was raised at a seaport and one of the specialties was like the exercise advised, with a slight exception. Along one of the piers was a board projection , and on this we would hang with the grip of fingers only, as explained. Under us was a ten-foot drop into the water. We would see how far along the ledge we could go before we finally dropped off. If you can locate a projecting ledge ledge you will be able to test the quality of your finger strength, and also check up on your progress.

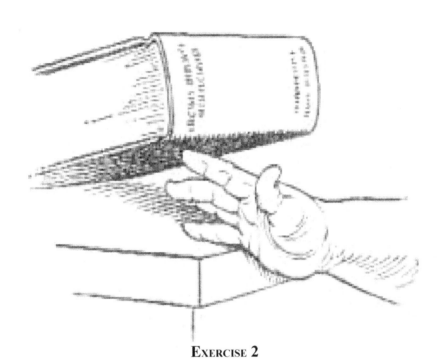

Exercise 2

EXERCISE THREE

Finger lifting is generally very popular with most people. In this exercise the forcep muscles of the hand are most strongly involved. It is a good stunt and a good exercise. When a person reaches the point where he can lift a 75-lb. disc of iron in the manner illustrated he is considered very strong indeed. The thickness of the disc generally used is 1 inch. Of course, I do not expect you to attempt 75 lbs. at first. It would be very foolish. Start out with a 25-lb. disc and commence by lifting it edgewise off the floor several times. In order to stimulate the finger gripping powers try the exercise out, first employing the index finger and thumb only; secondly, the thumb and the second finger only; next, employ only the thumb and third finger and lastly only the thumb and the little finger. From this stage you can progress employing two fingers and the thumb, using a heavier disc for the occasion, until finally you wind up the training period by making a grip lift using the entire hand as illustrated.

There is a difference in lifting the disc for exercise and lifting it to see how much weight you can raise off the floor. For exercise purposes it is permissible and advisable to bend the elbow and also the hand on the wrist in order to influence the wrist and arm muscles. This method, while better for grip and muscle development, would make a lift very difficult and decrease the poundage you could actually raise.

To lift, in a feat, the disc should be placed standing edgewise between the feet. The grip should fit over at the highest point of the disc to prevent rolling. Do not fit the thumb and fingers astride the disc so far as you can but leave a little space between the disc and the hand as shown. See that the arm is in a straight line hanging from the shoulder in a perpendicular line with the center of the disc. Grip *firmly but do not lift with the fingers*. Lift with the shoulder. The fingers must act only as the agents of pincer contact – the vise to hold and not to lift. Lift upward in a straight line by action of the shoulder and by slightly standing erect. With the non-lifting hand push hard upon the corresponding knee to produce poise and power.

In this stunt I have often walked with a 75-lb. disc suspended in the grip of each hand and have also snatched them to the shoulders in a clean movement.

An important point to remember in grips where the thumb is involved is to grip flatly with the thumb and finger, otherwise it has the same effect as pinching a ball between the fingers. You can so grip a ball between the fingers that the ball is forced out of the hand.

You will, I hope, still have in mind the value of making stunts out of these exercises. With this in mind you can handle the disc you have been exercising with in several different ways.

First practice spinning the plates. I don't mean to give it a twisting spin, but toss it in the air and catch it as it descends, allowing the swing to carry between the legs. Repeat this several times with each hand, then, as you toss with one hand, catch with the other. Thirdly, as you toss give the disc a quick pull as you let go so it revolves. You will find it more difficult to catch, but it will help to increase your finger strength.

Other ways of practice are to walk, holding the disc by the edge with the fingers. Walk with one in each hand also. Progress upon this by snatching the disc off the floor to the shoulder. As your gripping power increases snatch the disc to arm's length overhead. When you become very efficient snatch to arm's length overhead a disc in each hand.

As you do these stunts others will occur to you which you can practice in competition with your friends. Competition between friends makes for greater entertainment. You get on your mettle and in this way often bring physical abilities to the surface which you may otherwise have never known existed.

Mix fun with your training and it will become a real pleasure and the results will come quickly because you will stick at it longer and persevere more insistently.

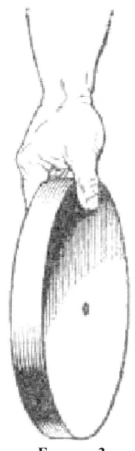

Exercise 3

EXERCISE FOUR

Here is a very old exercise and test of wrist strength. Years ago it was a very common test. It is to be regretted that we do not see more of it these days. One sure thing it will positively find the weak links in your hand, wrist and arm strength. At first practice with a broom alone. If this is too difficult when holding the end of the broom, merely move the hand down the handle and shorten the leverage. As you grow stronger move the hand grip toward the end. When this is accomplished progressively add a little weight by placing some small object on the straw end of the broom as shown. The picture illustrates an athlete raising a broom with a brick placed upon the straw end. When you become able to do this with a broom that has the regular length handle you can be well proud of your arm strength.

The broom must be in a straight line with the forearm and neither the elbow or arm must rest against or on the knee. The arm must act free and independent of any other aid or support.

A feat somewhat of this order was once a feature around blacksmith shops, the only difference being that they held sledge-hammers out in a straight line with the shoulder, grasping the handle of the sledge at the extreme end. Many a fellow with a strong wrist and forearm fell down on this stunt his deltoids or shoulder muscle were weak. Unfortunately there was no way of estimating the respective merits of these smiths with the brawny arms. Sledge hammers in the smithies varied from 6 pounds to 12 pounds, while the handle lengths and thicknesses were rarely alike. The length and thickness of the handle is of greater importance in this case than the weight. The shorter the handle the better the possibilities of performing the feat. The longer or the thicker the handle the more difficult it is.

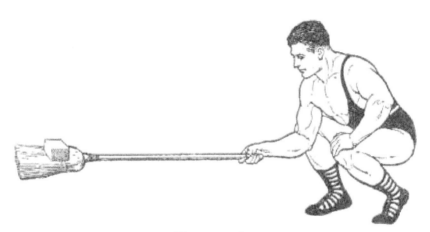

Exercise 4

As explained earlier in this book, Holtgrewe, of Cincinnati, was one of the strongest men America ever had and was remarkable with this broom and brick exercise. Others were Al Treloar, Joe Nordquest, Coulter and the wonderful Schmidt. The latter, while only a handful in body weight (about 126 lbs), was nigh invincible at gripping stunts.

When talking of famous strong men we must never omit Warren Lincoln Travis. He is beyond a doubt one of America's most colorful characters in the world of strength. His hand and finger strength is something to marvel at. In the years that have gone by he has been associated with all of the world's greatest strength athletes, and admire Travis for the great powers he has but never boast of.

At finger feats, hand and wrist feats, he is nigh invincible, and he is very clever. He possesses a wonderful knowledge of physical mechanics which aids him greatly in all the great feats he performs.

One of the feats Travis use to perform was to slide down a slanting wire suspended underneath the wire by a trapeze-like outfit, holding by the saddle with both hands a horse weighing around 600 or 700 lbs. It seems incredible, nevertheless it is true, such is the power of his hand grip.

Another character but very little known to the average American strength fan of today is Frank Fanks. Only a lightweight but with the strength of a first class heavyweight. His hands are as hard as steel from practicing his many difficult iron bending stunts.

EXERCISE FIVE

As I have remarked in this book, barrel lifting was very popular with the old-time strength athletes. For developing the fingers, hands, wrist and arms, there is nothing any better. Apart from this, barrel lifting is great for general body building. Of course, a barrel is not the handiest thing in the world to have around the house, but if a person is sincere in his search for great strength and muscular development he will always find a way to practice.

I wish to draw your attention to Exercise 5. this is purely a grip lifting exercise. Notice how the athlete is gripping the chines (the name applied to the edges of kegs and barrels). Practically speaking the only grip that can be secured is that given by the first joint of the fingers. The object is to keep the legs and the back straight and lift the barrel off the floor as high as you can. This done, replace the barrel on the floor and straighten out the fingers, then repeat the grip several times. When this is completed pass on Exercise 6.

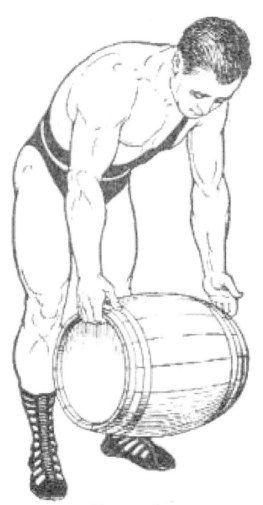

EXERCISE 5

EXERCISE SIX

In this case you lift the barrel up onto the thighs. This is the regular way to lift and carry a barrel. I have seen some men walk in this way carrying barrels weighing well over 300 lbs.

This calls for great strength in the legs as well as the fingers and arms. You just practice exercises five and six several times with a 100-lb. nail keg or barrel and you will be amazed at the results you get out of such practice.

Remember the instructions I have given you for carrying the barrel. This is very important.

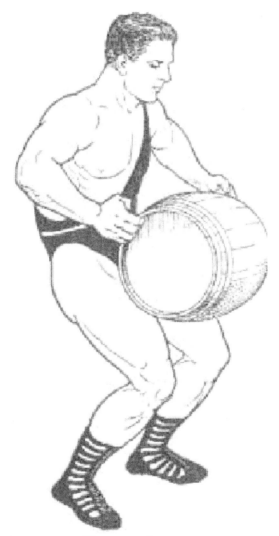

EXERCISE 6

EXERCISE SEVEN

Exercise 7 (a) shows the athlete with the barrel held at the shoulders. This is not so easy as it may at first appear. Great action of the arms and gripping muscles is necessary and a little practice will develop them to an extraordinary extent. The difficulty lies in getting the barrel to the shoulder, therefore it is very necessary that the exercise be first practiced with a small nail keg or an empty regular-sized barrel. If you employ a regular-sized barrel you will find it easier to manipulate it if you will pull the barrel in close to the body, then back, and thus aid the upward movement by allowing the barrel to roll up the body to the shoulders, Exercise 7 (a). From this point push the barrel to arm's length overhead as shown in Exercise 7 (b). This, in addition to developing great strength, will teach you equilibrium in lifting objects overhead as nothing else will.

There are several interesting ways of raising a barrel from the ground to arm's length overhead. One way is by what Swedish athletes term the "slow hang" position. That is, you lift the barrel off the ground slowly to the position as shown in Exercise 5. There you pause a moment and with a snap move to the position in Exercise 6 and from thence to the shoulder as in Exercise 7 (a), and arm's overhead as in Exercise 7 (b).

Another method is to pause as in Exercise 5 position and then in one movement sweep to the shoulders. This can be changed to sweeping the barrel from the ground to arm's length overhead or to the shoulders only. Another movement which will stimulate powerful forces is to pause at the point shown in Exercise 5 and then in one movement sweep the barrel to arm's length overhead.

Apart from the manner in which other muscles in the body will respond, the grip and the arms will obtain tremendous development through these exercises. You will not have to do much of this training before you will feel the results on the grip and in the arms. Man for man the old-time strength athlete was miles ahead of the present-day

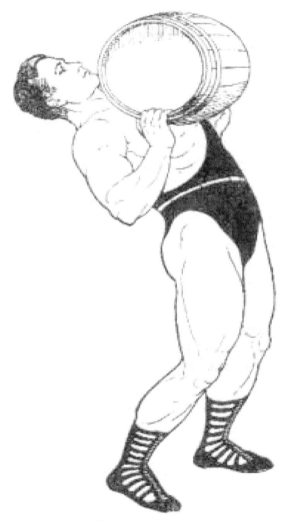

EXERCISE 7 (A)

athlete for grip. Rarely did one see a strength athlete of those days without a powerful and splendidly shaped pair of arms. The reason why we do not see so much grip and arm stunts today is because most of the crop of modern strength athletes are incapable. If they were equal to the tests they would perform them. A strong man is only bounded by the limitations of his own strength.

You should study carefully the illustrations accompanying these barrel exercises. I took great care when posing for them so that every detail would be caught by the artist. The finger grips and the hand positions are the most important, but overlook nothing. The stance of the legs, the position of the back and the distance when leaning back. The positions of the elbows are very important. Study them and you will find that progress will come faster to you in every way.

Here is an exercise which you have no doubt practiced a little in a slightly different way, but to practice it in the manner I shall now explain will call for a little courage.

Pull the barrel onto the thighs as in Exercise 6 and from this position quickly sit on the floor, straighten out the body and push the barrel to arm's length. Next, draw up the knees, lower the barrel onto them and quickly come to the erect position. A little practice with an empty barrel will soon overcome all the apparent difficulties of the stunt.

Another barrel feat is done when lying down flat on the back with the barrel laid on the floor behind the head. Reach over and grasp the chines of the barrel with the hands and pull the barrel over the head so that it rests on the hands, with arms supported by the elbows on the floor. From this position press the barrel to arm's length several times, then lower back behind the head and repeat the exercise over several times.* You will find this a dandy – an exercise you will like very much.

Some people are exceptionally clever at juggling barrels, but you want to be quite sure of yourself before you try them. Control of a barrel is easily lost and when it hits you, it does hit hard.

39

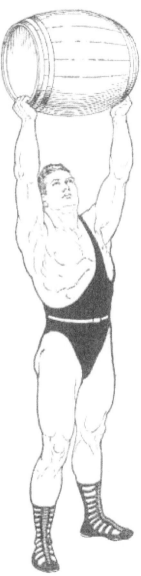

EXERCISE 7 (B)

Peter Zebbits – the Servian strong man – is an extraordinary performer with barrels. He can spin them and toss them, catching the barrel by the chines every time. No wonder he has such a phenomenal grip and a wrist that looks to be a writhing mass of thick, powerful, sinewy ligaments.

Such exercises, or feats, as I have described here require some skill to do them properly, but such skill is obtained through practice. You will get real satisfaction and pleasure from your efforts, however, and will be well rewarded for the time you spend on these exercises. This is equally true of the Exercise Eight which follows.

EXERCISE EIGHT

A very difficult exercise is that of shouldering a barrel with one hand. If you asked the average fellow to do this stunt he would be stumped to know how to go about it. It is an exercise feat that requires speed, strength and perfect poise. The many muscular changes the body goes through in this process are remarkable. Some fellows are decidedly clever and strong in manipulating the barrel to one shoulder. To commence, the barrel must be rocked forward so that it is balanced on the front edge. The knee should next be inserted under the nearest edge of the barrel. Grasp the barrel and with a powerful back and arm pull, pull the barrel toward the body and at the same time toss up with the knee as shown in Exercise 8 (a). Then immediately let go with the gripping hand and catch the barrel as it travels to the body within the fold of the elbow. From this point, by leaning sharply sideways the barrel will roll onto the shoulder as shown in Exercise 8 (b). This may seem like a lot to remember but if you practice with an empty barrel you will soon master the changes. The thing to do is to memorize well the changes before you do them and then work fast, especially after the barrel is being pulled to the knee and tossed. Loise Cyr, the great French-Canadian athlete, frequently shouldered with one hand a barrel filled with beer that weighed nearly 400 lbs.

Lifting a barrel with water in it is very difficult unless the barrel is completely filled. A great teat was to half fill it with a mixture of sand and water. The way it would slop around made the handling of it twice as hard.

Before I close those barrel exercises I would like to give you one more. When you have gotten the barrel to the shoulders, whether to one shoulder as in Exercise 8 (b) or both, as in Exercise 7 (a), transfer it to one hand. In order to do this you must steady the barrel with one hand and manipulate the barrel so it is seated on the palm of the lifting hand. The barrel should be pointing back and front as in Exercise 8 (b). From that position steadily push the barrel to arm's length, but first see that the balance is perfect. A barrel is the meanest thing in the world once you lose control of it.

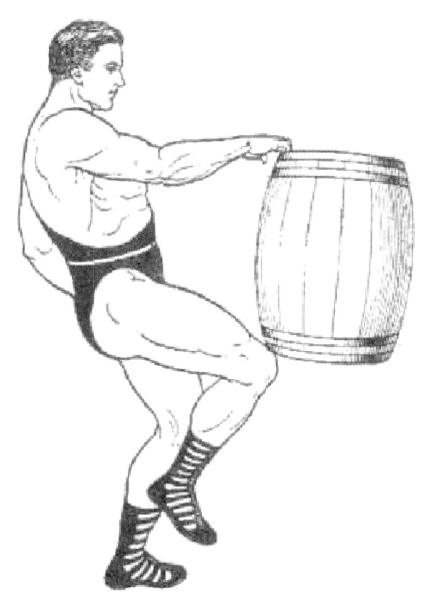

EXERCISE 8 (A)

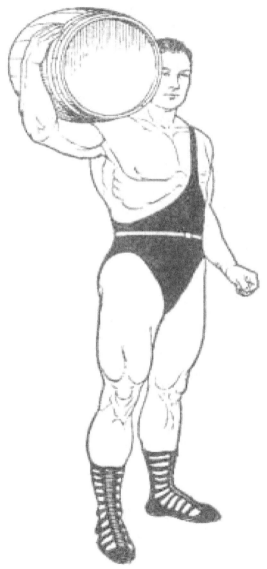

EXERCISE 8 (B)

In conclusion, let me say, do not neglect any of these exercises or omit them from your training schedule. They will repay you more quickly than any other form of grip exercise, with the exception of block weight and kettle bell juggling, which is nothing more or less than a contributory variation of what I have explained here. Barrel stunting is beyond a doubt the supreme test of you grip strength. It will build it for you to a marvelous degree. The power of your fingers, the forcep power of the thumb, the strength of the hands, wrists and forearms will increase almost from your first practice period. You will indeed get that grip of steel which we all so much admire and desire. Practice on these exercises will develop the forearm muscles which would not respond to any other form of exercise. From shoulder to finger tips you will be the proud owner of a mighty arm and will have in each hand the vice-like crushing grip of a steel bear-trap. By such practice you may become a Pedley, Marx, Saxon, Vanstitart, Travis, Fanks or a Coulter. It is not impossible. It is simply up to you – now you have been shown how.

For more old time classics of strength, visit:

STRONGMANBOOKS.COM

Currently Available:

The Development of Physical Power by Arthur Saxon

Text Book of Weight Lifting by Arthur Saxon

Bob Hoffman's Simplified System of Barbell Training

Muscle Control by Maxick

System of Physical Training by Eugene Sandow

York Hand Balancing Courses 1 & 2

The Way to Live by George Hackenschmidt

How to Learn Muscle Control by Otto Arco and Alan Calvert

Molding Mighty Men Series by George Jowett

More coming soon...

Made in the USA
Las Vegas, NV
14 August 2023

76098422R00030